Linda T. Williams

Fight The Sugar Addiction : Low Carb and Sugar-Free recipes ideas

A Short Guide to Fight Efficiently Sugar Addiction Withdrawal Symptoms

Books on Demand

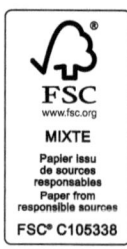

© 2019 by Linda T. Williams
Edition : Books on Demand, 12/14, Rond-Point des Champs-Elysées, 75008 Paris (France)
Impression : Books on Demand GmbH, Norderstedt, (Germany).
ISBN : 9782322133383
Legal deposit : february 2019
All rights reserved.

Introduction

Sugar is the generic name for sweet-tasting, soluble carbohydrates, many of which are used in food. There are various types of sugar derived from different sources. Simple sugars are called monosaccharides and include glucose (also known as dextrose), fructose, and galactose. The "table sugar" or "granulated sugar" most customarily used as food is sucrose, a disaccharide of glucose and fructose. Sugar is used in prepared foods (e.g., cookies and cakes) and is added to some foods and beverages (e.g., coffee and tea). In the body, sucrose is hydrolysed into the simple sugars fructose and glucose. Other disaccharides include maltose from malted grain, and lactose from milk. Longer chains of sugars are called oligosaccharides or polysaccharides. Some other chemical substances, such as glycerol and sugar alcohols may also have a sweet taste, but are not classified as sugars. Diet foodsubstitutes for sugar include aspartame and sucralose, a chlorinated derivative of sucrose. Sugars are found in the tissues of most plants and are present in sugarcane and sugar beet in sufficient concentrations for efficient commercial extraction. In 2017–18, the world production of sugar was 185 million tonnes. The average person consumes about 24 kilograms (53 lb) of sugar each year (33.1 kg in developed countries), equivalent to over 260 food calories per person per day. Since the latter part of the twentieth century, it has been questioned whether a diet high in sugars, especially refined sugars, is good for human health. Over-consumption of sugar has been implicated in the occurrence of obesity, diabetes, cardiovascular disease, dementia, and tooth decay. Numerous studies have been undertaken to try to clarify the position, but with varying results, mainly because of the difficulty of finding populations for use as controls that do not consume or are largely free of any sugar consumption. It's no secret that governments all over the world are starting to crack down on sugar. They are passing taxes on sugary drinks and snacks, banning them from schools, and more treatment programs are becoming open to people who believe they are addicted to sugar. But what is the truth? Is sugar the new enemy?

The Different Types of Sugar

Coca leaves were used for centuries in their natural state to chew on or to make tea. This was normal and there were no issues. But, then they were highly processed and turned into a dangerous and addictive drug known as cocaine.

The innocent poppy flower suffered the same fate. Formerly a safe and effective tea, often used for relaxation and pain, it got super-processed and became a powerful, dangerous and addictive opiate.

Sugar first starts out as sugar cane - a healthy stalking plant. Used in its natural form you can't consume enough to make you sick. But super-concentrated and processed it becomes like a drug. In fact, with lab rats, sugar outperformed cocaine as the drug of choice.

It's important to know that there are various types of sugar, some natural and some very processed - to the point that even if they started natural, they are no longer natural.

- **Fructose** – Don't get confused by the word. While fructose is derived from fruit, it's gone through processing that makes it a highly-concentrated form of sugar. This type of fructose should really be called "industrial fructose". Eating fructose from natural fruit is not unsafe and should not be avoided. Once processed, though, it becomes something else entirely and causes a lot of health problems.

- **Glucose** – This is sugar that's in your blood. You get it from natural plant foods such as carbohydrates, fruits, and vegetables, especially starchy ones. It's one of the most important medications and very readily available in nature. It supplies almost all the energy to the brain. It's important for metabolic health, respiration and more. If you want to be able to think clearly, you must have the right amount of glucose. Glucose is created industrially by using starchy plants like corn, rice, wheat, and other ingredients.

- **Lactose** – Found in milk, it's made from galactose and glucose. Industrially it's produced as a by-product of the dairy industry. Most humans produce lactase to help digest this type of sugar far into adulthood. But some people, especially from eastern and south-eastern Asia and some parts of Africa cannot properly digest this type of sugar in adulthood.

- **Maltose** – This sugar is found in the germination process as the seeds break down their starch stores for food to sprout and grow. This type of sugar can cause many intolerances as well as weight gain, kidney stones and more. However, eating it in its natural form such as in sweet potatoes, soybeans, barley and wheat (other than those who suffer from celiac) is healthy.

- **Sucrose** – This type of sugar comes from cane and beets. Modern processing can make it look just like table sugar. Before it's been processed it has a lot of health benefits, vitamins, and minerals. Honey is mostly fructose and glucose with trace amounts of sucrose.

As you see, most sugars start in a very natural state and aren't bad in their natural and most whole form until they undergo super-processing. It's the super-processing that's bad for you, because it makes natural sugars into highly addictive drug-like substances.

Forms and uses

- Rock candy crystallized out of a supersaturated sugar solution that contains green dye.
- Brown sugars are granulated sugars, either containing residual molasses, or with the grains deliberately coated with molasses to produce a light- or dark-colored sugar. They are used in baked goods, confectionery, and toffees.
- Granulated sugars are used at the table, to sprinkle on foods and to sweeten hot drinks (coffee and tea), and in home baking to add sweetness and texture to baked products (cookies and cakes) and desserts (pudding and ice cream). They are also used as a preservative to prevent micro-organisms from growing and perishable food from spoiling, as in candied fruits, jams, and marmalades.
- Invert sugars and syrups are blended to manufacturers specifications and are used in breads, cakes, and beverages for adjusting sweetness, aiding moisture retention and avoiding crystallization of sugars.
- Liquid sugars are strong syrups consisting of 67% granulated sugar dissolved in water. They are used in the food processing of a wide range of products including beverages, hard candy, ice cream, and jams.
- Low-calorie sugars and artificial sweeteners are often made of maltodextrin with added sweeteners. Maltodextrin is an easily digestible synthetic polysaccharide consisting of short chains of glucose molecules and is made by the partial hydrolysis of starch. The added sweeteners are often aspartame, saccharin, stevia, or sucralose.
- Milled sugars (known as confectioner's sugar and powdered sugar) are ground to a fine powder. They are used as powdered sugar (also known as icing sugar or confectionary sugar), for dusting foods and in baking and confectionery.

- Molasses is commonly used to make rum, and sugar byproducts are used to make ethanol for fuel.
- Polyols are sugar alcohols and are used in chewing gums where a sweet flavor is required that lasts for a prolonged time in the mouth.
- Screened sugars are crystalline products separated according to the size of the grains. They are used for decorative table sugars, for blending in dry mixes and in baking and confectionery.
- Sugar cubes (sometimes called sugar lumps) are white or brown granulated sugars lightly steamed and pressed together in block shape. They are used to sweeten drinks.
- Sugarloaf was the usual cone-form in which refined sugar was produced and sold until the late 19th century. This shape is still in use in Germany (for preparation of Feuerzangenbowle), in Iran and Morocco.
- Syrups and treacles are dissolved invert sugars heated to develop the characteristic flavors. (Treacles have added molasses.) They are used in a range of baked goods and confectionery including toffees and licorice.
- In winemaking, fruit sugars are converted into alcohol by a fermentation process. If the must formed by pressing the fruit has a low sugar content, additional sugar may be added to raise the alcohol content of the wine in a process called chaptalization. In the production of sweet wines, fermentation may be halted before it has run its full course, leaving behind some residual sugar that gives the wine its sweet taste.

13 Reasons Sugar Is Bad for You

Let's look at many of the reasons sugar is thought to be bad for you. Some people say it's one of the worst things you can introduce to your system, even above fat.

1. **Your Immune System** – If you consume too much processed sugar you can reduce your ability to kill germs inside your body. It doesn't take much, either. Just two sodas can stop the ability to fight off that flu bug and lead to falling ill. This doesn't mean you shouldn't get vaccines if you don't eat sugar, but when it comes to health, including dental health, avoiding added sugar can boost your immunity exponentially.

2. **Mineral Balance** – If you have trouble sleeping at night, are constipated and having other problems, you could be having trouble with your mineral balance. If you eat a lot of sugar, you are likely depleting your magnesium stores to process all of it. Plus, you will lose more chromium through your urine if you eat a lot of sugar.

3. **Behavior Problems** – Every parent on the planet will tell you that sugar and lack of sugar can affect their child's behavior. If a child is hungry and their blood sugar is low, they will be sleepy and grumpy. If a child has an overdose of sugar, they will become agitated and animated. The key to better behavior is blood sugar balance.

4. **Empty Calories** – The fact is, processed sugar has no health benefits whatsoever. Therefore, when you eat sugary meals, you're eating empty calories that will cause weight gain. The fact that sugar is often combined with fat and salt will make the effects even worse. It's better to avoid added sugar when you can.

5. **Elevated Insulin Responses** – When your insulin response is healthy, your cells will release the right

amount of insulin. But, if you regularly consume sugar, especially in "overdose" amounts, your body will become confused about when to release insulin and when not to.

6. **Damages Cells and Tissues** – The tissue in your eyes, kidneys, nerves and more seem to carry sugar a lot longer than other organs. This means that the body can suffer damage from that remaining sugar because it damages small blood vessels.

7. **Causes High Blood Triglyceride Levels** – There are no symptoms for high blood triglyceride levels. The only way to know if you have high triglycerides is by getting a blood test. It's usually part of your overall cholesterol test.

8. **Contributes to Hyperactivity** – There are studies that show both results. Sugar does cause hyperactivity and sugar doesn't cause it. You must remember that any drug can affect one human one way, and another human another way. But, parents often report problems with hyperactivity in their child after consuming too much sugar. You can't ignore the possibility.

9. **Anxiety** – Refined sugars enter the blood stream quickly, and leave the blood stream quickly. This process can manifest in more anxiety overall. Even though often people who are addicted to sugar eat to suppress anxiety, it's just making the problem much worse. It's best to avoid added sugars in the first place.

10. **Poor Concentration** – Again, the reason sugar may affect concentration is because of the speed by which processed sugar can invade blood cells and then leave them. You need a balanced level of glucose to feed your brain, not short bursts of sugar such as in the form of soft drinks or cereal.

11. **Feeds Some Cancers** – The fact is, cancer cells love sugar. That's because like most living things they need sugar to grow. But, not all sugars are created equal. Cancer cells love white sugar, white flour, and high fructose corn syrup. The good thing is that if you simply reduce your consumption of processed sugar, you can cut your cancer risks.

12. **Hypoglycemia** – Low blood sugar happens in people who have a condition called hypoglycemia. This can be a condition on its own, but it can also happen in people who have diabetes and take medications like insulin because their bodies don't produce enough on their own.

13. **Poor Digestion** – Processed sugar is very acidic. The more alkaline you can make your body, the healthier you'll become. If you have an acidic stomach you'll suffer from heartburn, GERD, and other digestion problems.

Each person is affected differently. It's best to look at your own symptoms and health issues and if you have any of these problems, try eliminating processed sugar first to see if you notice any changes in your health.

The Surprising Places Sugar Hides

The hidden sugar in our diet is hard to find. You'll be amazed at the things that have added and often unnecessary sugar inside.

- **Breakfast Cereal** – Most of you could have guessed this one, but we're not talking about the sugar in sugary cereal. We're talking about hidden sugar in so-called healthy cereals. Some "healthy" cereals have more than 23 grams of sugar per serving.

- **Asian Food** – Most restaurant-made or packaged Asian food has an enormous amount of sugar in it. Even sushi. The way you make sushi rice includes adding sugar to it. You can make your own Asian food to ensure that the sugar level is not too high.

- **Canned and Packaged Soups and Sauces** – Thankfully, all you have to do is check the labels. Some yogurt has more than 15 grams of sugar! Even spaghetti sauce and gravy can have more sugar than a soda pop. If you want to be sure to eat less sugar, read labels and find no-sugar options or make your own.

- **Frozen Yogurt** – Just because the word yogurt is in it doesn't mean it's healthy. It's just as sugary as regular ice-cream. It's a dessert. Treat it as if it's a dessert. Don't use it for a meal, and don't believe you're eating healthier. If you prefer real ice cream for a snack you are now free to eat it instead, as one is not better than the other when it comes to sugar.

- **Smoothies** – They're all the rage and there are many smoothie shops out there banking on it. But, most smoothie shops use fruit with added sugar which removes any benefits you would have from drinking a smoothie at all. If you make your own, watch it when recipes ask for dried fruit too. Using whole, fresh fruit is much better.

- **Bread** – While there is some bread that is good for you, most bread is made with highly refined flour and sugar. Both of these affect blood sugar. Even wheat bread may be high in sugar, so you need to read the labels. Bread that is usually low in sugar is rye or spelt. Plus, you can make your own to avoid additives and sugar that can harm your health.

- **Condiments** – You know we all like to dip everything. But, if you dip your fresh apples or celery into the wrong thing, you may be making matters worse. Instead, make your own condiments or read the labels. Today there are many low-sugar varieties of condiments, including low-sugar ketchup.

- **Canned Beans** – Check the labels on canned beans, especially ones with any type of sauce on them like chili beans or baked beans. These are usually so high in sugar that if you compared it to a cake you wouldn't know which was which just by the amount of sugar.

- **Muffins** – You probably already realize that some muffins are high in sugar, but even the ones that sound healthy are just cakes in muffin form with a healthy flour or healthy name added. They are all high in sugar. There are some recipes for low-sugar muffins, though; just search the net and you're sure to find them. You don't have to do without.

- **Yogurt** – Just like frozen yogurt is high in sugar, so is most sweetened yogurt - including low-fat yogurt. The best way to combat this problem is to make your own yogurt or eat yogurt as a dessert. You can also buy plain yogurt and add your own fruit and stevia to create a low-sugar snack that is healthy due to the probiotics in yogurt.

The lesson is that anything premade and packaged is in danger of having too much sugar. It's best to read the labels and judge for yourself. Keep in mind that the average adult should not consume more than 90 grams, or 5 percent of their total calories, in added sugar daily.

How Much Sugar Is Too Much?

One thing that needs to be clear is that there is a difference from naturally occurring sugars and added sugar. There is sugar in all plant food and plant food is good for you. In fact, most of your plate should make up plant food if you want to be at your optimum health.

So, it breaks down that adults should not consume more than about 90 grams in total of all sugars each day. How much of that constitutes added sugar depends on your ideal daily caloric intake.

That means if you eat 1500 calories each day, you can eat 90 grams of sugar a day. How much of that you want to be processed and added sugar is up to you. But obviously, keeping the amount of added sugar lower is better for your health. This gives you some room to experiment with your health and to have a little fun on your birthday.

When you consider that a cup of grapes has 15 grams of sugar but a can of coke has 39 grams, it makes the choice easier. If you really want a drink, you can try a sugar-free Zevia or even better, LaCroix. But a tall glass of filtered water with a cup of grapes will fill you up longer. The main thing is to find substitutes that you truly enjoy and like, while not overshooting the 90 grams of sugar allowance you have for each day.

The more natural sugars that you consume within that 90 grams, the healthier you'll feel. And there are many low glycemic choices that you can make.

Fruit

- Apples – 1 small = 15g
- Apricots – 1 cup = 15g

- Banana – 1 medium = 14g
- Blackberries – 1 cup whole = 7g
- Blueberries – 1 cup whole = 15g
- Cantaloupe – 1 cup diced = 12g
- Cranberries – 1 cup whole = 4g
- Grapefruit – 1 cup = 16g
- Guavas – 1 cup = 15g
- Honeydew – 1 cup diced = 14g
- Lemons – 1 wedge = 0.2g
- Limes - 1 wedge = 0.15g
- Papaya – 1 cup 1" cubed = 11g
- Peaches – 1 cup sliced = 13g
- Raspberries – 1 cup whole = 5g
- Rhubarb – 1 cup diced = 1.3g
- Strawberries – 1 cup whole = 7g
- Tomatoes – 1 large whole = 4.8g
- Watermelon – 1 cup diced = 9g

Vegetables

- Artichokes – 1 large = 1.6g
- Asparagus – 1 cup = 2.5g
- Broccoli – 1 cup chopped = 1.5g
- Carrots – 1 medium = 2.9g
- Celery – 1 cup chopped = 1.8g
- Corn – 1 cup = 1.1g
- Cucumber – 1 8-in = 5g
- Green Beans – 1 cup = 3.3g
- Kale – 1 cup chopped = 1.6g
- Lettuce – 1 head = 2.8g
- Soybean sprouts – 1 cup = 0.1g
- Spinach – 1 cup = 0.1g
- Summer squash – 1 cup sliced = 2.5g
- Swiss chard – 1 cup = 0.4g

As you can see, most natural foods don't really have "too much" sugar. If you can eat 90 grams of sugar a day and you choose wisely from the lower sugar fruits and veggies, you'll be surprised at how much you can eat if you avoid added sugars. When you consider that one teaspoon of processed sugar is 4.2 grams, you can decide what is best to eat in every given situation.

Are You Addicted to Sugar?

As you read this report, do you start thinking about ways to get around the 90-gram maximum of sugar that you can have each day? Note that the 90 grams of sugar (per UK government guidelines) you can consume per day has nothing to do with how many carbohydrates you eat each day. This is a separate number that you should be tracking.

Here are some common behaviors that predict sugar addition:

- **You Eat Too Much** – If there are some foods that you just can't stop eating, assume they're likely high in sugar. Sugar doesn't really make you satiated, so it's hard to stop. This is made worse if sugar is combined with sodium and fat. For example, you may be eating donuts which are also high in salt and fat, but would you really eat them without the sugar? Doubtful.

- **You Crave Processed Carbohydrates** – If you're often craving refined carbs like chips, crackers, and bread, then you may just have a problem with sugar. Often, eliminating added sugars can reduce cravings that you're having for high processed carbs over time.

- **You Crave Salty Foods** – With processed foods, salt and sugar go together very well. If you feel like you could lick a salt lick and be happy, you may be addicted to sugar.

Look at the amount of sugar in the snacks you normally eat. If they're highly processed, you can bet they have too much added sugar.

- **You Crave Meat** – This might seem strange, but if you crave meat when you really don't need it and aren't really that hungry, you may really be craving the spices that are often on meat such as wing sauce which is very high in sugar.

- **Every Meal Is High in Sugar** – Is your typical meal higher in sugar than it should be? Keep in mind that the maximum of 90 grams is a maximum. It doesn't mean you need to eat that much sugar. If you feel bad and aren't healthy, you can always cut that amount down. The best way to do that is avoid added sugars and only eat sugar that is naturally in plants.

- **You Get Moody without Sugar** – If you find that you are often feeling grumpy and moody, the problem might sugar. If you often suffer dips and rises in blood sugar, when you have a dip you will suffer from grumpy moods. This can be exacerbated by eating sugary things like candy which will provide a fast jump and a quick fall.

- **You Feel Powerless Over Sugar** – Do you ever feel like you don't even want to eat that sugary snack but you do it anyway because you know it'll make you feel better? This is common in people who work long days; students especially. It's true that eating a sugary snack will help temporarily, but you'd do far better eating a fruit snack with only natural sugars and fiber to help slow down the sugar absorption.

- **You Start and End Your Day with Sugar** – Look at your entire day. What do you eat in the morning? What do you eat before bed? What is the first and last thing you eat each day? If you're eating sugar in the morning and at night, especially added processed sugar and not sugar in whole plants, then that is a sign that you may have an addiction to sugar.

- **You Suffer a 3 PM Slump** – If you work in an office, you'll notice this a lot more than if you are retired or work from home. But pay attention if somewhere after lunch you start falling asleep while you're working or feel as if you need a nap. Look at your diet. Are you giving yourself energy for lunch or are you setting yourself up for a sugar crash?

If you are going through any of these issues, it is wise to calculate how much sugar you're eating in any given day. Most people eat double the sugar maximum of 90 grams a day due to added and processed sugars, including hidden sugars.

Tips for Breaking Your Sugar Habit

Thankfully, you don't need to work that hard to break your sugar addiction. It's only hard if you shoot for zero sugar. That would not be healthy. Instead, first just shoot for a reduction, and then cut it back more and more through solid food choices.

- **Avoid Processed Food** – The biggest culprit when it comes to sugar in food is processed food. Processed food has tons of sugar and if it doesn't, it has tons of chemicals. Avoiding processed food can eliminate almost all of the added sugar you're eating.

- **Get Plenty of Sunshine** – It might seem weird, but one reason people like to eat sugar is serotonin, the feel-good hormone. When you eat a lot of sugar you'll get a spike in serotonin. Of course, you also get a crash. There are better ways to increase serotonin levels; one is the sunshine. Of course, you'll also get vitamin D which can also improve your mood.

- **Get Plenty of Sleep** – If you have trouble sleeping at night, then you need to get to the root cause of why. Avoid sugars, caffeine, and anything stimulating two to three hours before bed. You should go to sleep on an empty stomach for the best sleep.

- **Drink Enough Water** – Staying hydrated is important to avoid any type of cravings, including sugar cravings. When you're born, you have a perfect thirst detector. But, life often causes us to deny our bodies' signals. Therefore, measure your water to ensure that you're drinking a minimum of 64 ounces to 100 ounces of water a day depending upon your weight.

- **Focus on Stability** – You want to try to keep your sugar balanced. One way to do that is to have regular meal times. For you, that may be six meals a day; for others than will end up being the traditional three meals a day. It depends on what works best for you. You should eat when you feel real hunger pangs.

- **Eat Your Greens** – For some reason, when you eat more greens like turnip greens, spinach, kale and so forth, your sweet cravings will go away. So, instead of eating something sweet when you get the craving, try eating a bowl of steamed spinach with good red wine vinegar on it and your cravings will disappear.

- **Incorporate Fermented Foods and Drinks** – Not only are they good to help keep your stomach acid and bacteria balanced, fermented foods and drinks are also great sweet tooth killers. You can buy prepared fermented foods or make your own. Keep in mind a very small amount of sugar is used in fermentation, but that is okay.

- **Meditate** – Sometimes sugar cravings are just a sign that you need to slow down and center yourself. Stress can play a huge part in appetite and cravings. Take the time to meditate, at least 10 minutes per day. If you don't want to meditate, prayer or sitting silently also works.

Incorporating these tips into your day can make a huge difference when you're trying to end sugar cravings and break your sugar habit. Remember that it's not going to happen overnight either. Just focus on adding in good things to your life rather than on what you're eliminating.

How to Fight Sugar Addiction Withdrawal Symptoms

When you first embark on eliminating added sugar from your diet, you're going to experience some withdrawal symptoms - especially if some of your sugary treats included caffeine. You don't want to use a bunch of fake things to sub for sugar, so it's best to try to get over each symptom you have.

- **Depression** – If you notice after giving up added sugar you're feeling depressed, ensure that you are eating some natural sugars like those found in fruit and veggies. You don't want to have zero carbohydrates. Carbohydrates make you feel good. Just eat them without added sugar, oil and fat.

- **A headache** – This is more than likely caused from drinking less caffeine. But, if you do find that you're getting headaches, check your hydration. If you were used to sugary drinks, it can be hard to drink plain water. But, it's imperative that you drink enough each day.

- **Anxiety** – Anxiety manifests itself in many ways to different people. Some people get a fluttery feeling in their stomach. Others experience shortness of breath or heart palpitations. It can be very severe in some people. If you find that you're experiencing a lot of anxiety, the best thing to do is go to your doctor for a blood test. Some illnesses like hypothyroid which has nothing to do with sugar restriction can cause anxiety. Otherwise, just check your hydration level, sleep level, and ensure that you're eating enough calories for your ideal weight.

- **Irritable Mood** – Feeling moody? When your blood sugar gets too low you can feel moody. This can be remedied by eating more often. Try to balance your meals with the right amounts of protein, fat, and carbohydrates for your personal needs. Don't allow yourself to get too hungry; this is a sure-fire way to end up feeling moody. Keep healthy snacks around like apples and no sugar added peanut butter.

- **Fatigue** – Still feeling that 3 pm slump? Feeling tired and foggy all the time? This is a sign that you're not eating enough carbohydrates. Remember that veggies are good carbs and you should eat them in plentiful amounts. It can also mean that you need to drink more water.

- **Achy Muscles** – This is one of the first signs of dehydration. A lot of people who used to drink sugary drinks for most of their hydration find it difficult to get enough water. Drink at least eight glasses of water a day. For snacks, eat hydrating food like apples, carrots, oranges and other fresh fruit and veggies.

- **Cravings** – When you notice you're getting super-strong sugar cravings, it's time to look at your list of things to do during cravings. You can still eat something sweet, but instead of candy or processed food, pick something fresh like a bowl of berries or sliced apples.

The symptoms of sugar withdrawal are more difficult for some people than others. Be patient with yourself. If you cave in and eat processed sugar, drink extra water, move more, and be prepared next time with a healthy snack. Don't forget to try the greens and vinegar.

Recipe Ideas to Keep Your Sugar Cravings at Bay

One way to avoid eating too much sugar is to be ready. If you're prepared with food to eat when you have a craving, when you're feeling tired, and when you're hungry, you'll do a lot better sticking to your goals.

Frozen Fruit Dessert

This isn't as much of a recipe as an idea. You can use your food processor, high-speed blender, magic bullet or a gadget like the Yonana Frozen Healthy Dessert Maker (http://amzn.to/2jyNk2w). All you do is freeze the fruit you want to use for a while, then feed it through the Yonana or blend it in one of the blenders or the food processor. It's simple and tastes wonderful. Tip: Use the ripest fruit you can for the sweetest flavor.

Snacks

The best snacks have a good balance of fat and protein. These low-sugar snack ideas will help you if you miss sugar at all.

Apples and Peanut Butter – Skip the bread and just slice up an apple, then spread it with sugar-free peanut butter. The best peanut butter has one ingredient. Peanuts. The fiber in the apple makes the sugar digest slowly. The fat and protein in the peanut butter keep you satiated.

Fiber Rich Loaf – Everyone likes bread but it can pack a huge sugar punch. But, you can make your own fiber-rich bread that is low in sugar and healthy for you.

No Sugar Fiber Loaf

1 cup hulled, salt-free raw pumpkin seeds
1/2 cup hemp seeds
1/2 cup raw peeled almonds
1.5 cup rolled oats
2 tbsp chia seeds
3 tbsp psyllium husk powder
1 tsp fine grain sea salt
1 tbsp honey
3 tbsp apple sauce
1.5 cup water

Combine all dry ingredients. Set aside. Combine all wet ingredients in a separate bowl. Then pour the wet ingredients into the dry. Mix until it forms a thick dough. If you notice that it's too dry, you can add more water. Form into a dough and put into a prepared bread pan. You can prepare your bread pan with some oil spread on with a paper towel, or you can line the pan with parchment paper.

Cover pan and dough with a towel and let sit in a warm place for at least two hours. When the dough has risen enough, you'll know because it keeps its shape when you touch it lightly with your finger.

Bake in a 350-degree F oven on the middle rack for about 30 to 40 minutes. Done bread will sound hollow when thumped.

Fermented Veggies

Let's make this simple. You can chop a bunch of veggies, or you can go to the fresh section of your grocery and buy prechopped veggies in bags, or from the salad bar. It's up to you how you do it. But, you'll want to chop them smaller anyway. Probably 1/2 inch pieces will work best.

In addition, you need some glass jars with sealable lids, such as canning jars.

Chop a mixture of veggies that you enjoy. Include at least a couple of apples or carrots due to the sweet flavor they provide. Add some ginger too if you like the flavor. Sprinkle all with salt.

Fill each jar with your mixture of chopped veggies tightly. Leave one inch of space from the top. Smash the veggies into the jar. You want them very tight. Then into each filled jar, put the following mixture into the jar until it's one inch below the top.

Brine

4 cups water
1 tbsp sea salt

Mix until the salt is totally dissolved.

Ensure that the veggie mixture always stays under the water in the jar. If you need to, weight the mixture down with a stone or weight. Cover with some cheesecloth and a rubber band. Keep in a warm spot for three to five days.

Check the mixture daily to ensure that everything stays under the brine. You'll know when your fermented veggies are done when your veggies are bubbling. That shows that the fermenting process has completed. Your veggies should also smell a little sour but you should like the smell. They should also taste good. After that has happened, put the normal lids the jars on and put in the fridge.

sugar free recipes without sugar substitutes

LOW CARB CHOCOLATE CHIP SKILLET COOKIE

Prep Time 15 minutes Cook Time 40 minutes Total Time 55 minutes Servings 12 Calories 267 kcal

Ingredients

3/4 cup butter softened

4 oz cream cheese softened

4 oz sour cream

1 cup Sukrin Gold

1 tsp vanilla extract

1/2 tsp vanilla liquid stevia

1/4 cup heavy cream

2 eggs

2 cups sesame flour (216 grams) or if no tree nut allergies use almond flour

1 tsp xanthan gum

1 tsp baking powder

1 tsp salt

1/2 cup sugar free chocolate chips

Instructions

Preheat the oven to 350 degrees F.

Add your butter, cream cheese, sour cream to a stand mixer and blend until smooth.

Add the sweetener, vanilla extract, stevia and milk to the mixer and blend until combined. Taste and adjust sweetener if needed.

Add the remaining ingredients to the mixer, except the chocolate chips. Blend until incorporated then stir in the chocolate chips by hand.

Grease a 9 inch cast iron skillet and spread the batter into the skillet.

Bake for 30- 40 minutes or until a toothpick in center comes out clean.

Remove from oven and allow to cool for 20-30minutes before serving.

SUGAR-FREE PALEO PECAN SNOWBALL COOKIES

Prep Time 5 minutes Cook Time 15 minutes Total Time 20 minutes Servings 24 Calories 112 kcal

Ingredients

8 tbsp Ghee or use butter if not paleo

1 1/2 cup almond flour 150 grams

1 cup pecans 120 grams, chopped

1/2 cup Swerve Confectioners Sweetener 78 grams

1 tsp vanilla extract

1/2 tsp vanilla liquid stevia

1/4 tsp salt

extra confectioners to roll balls in

Instructions

Preheat oven to 350 degrees F.

Place all ingredients into food processor and process until batter forms a ball. Pulse if needed.

Taste batter, adjust sweetener if needed.

Line a baking sheet with silpat or parchment.

Use a cookie scoop and make 24 mounds.

Roll each mound in the palm of your hand.

Place in freezer for 20-30 minutes.

Place in oven for 15 minutes or until golden around edges.

Allow to cool slightly.

Once able to handle roll each in some confectioners sweetener.

Allow to cool completely before storing in an air tight container.

Recipe Notes

Net Carbs: 1g

Healthy Chocolate Pancakes

These gluten-free chocolate pancakes will feed your brunch obsession. Topped with fresh fruit, crunchy buckwheat groats and a decadent melted chocolate, the whole fam will love these delicious morsels!

Ingredients

2 eggs.

1 cup milk of your choice (full-fat, almond, oat, rice).

3/4 cups buckwheat flour.

1 cup almond meal.

1/4 cup raw cacao powder.

1 teaspoon rice malt syrup.

1 teaspoon baking powder.

Butter or coconut oil, for frying.

Serving

50 g dark chocolate, melted.

100 g strawberries, hulled and sliced.

1/4 cup cacao nibs.

Instructions

1. Place eggs and milk in a large mixing bowl. Whisk together.

2. Add almond meal, buckwheat flour, cacao and baking powder into the mixing bowl. Stir mixture with a wooden spoon until smooth.

3. Heat a large frypan over low-medium heat. Grease the pan with a little butter and add in ¼ cup of mixture per pancake. Cook for 2–3 minutes until bubbles appear on the surface, then flip and cook for another one minute.

4. Place pancakes onto an ovenproof dish and place into an oven on 140°C/275°F/Gas Mark 1 to stay warm while you cook the remaining pancakes.

5. Serve pancakes with your choice of toppings.

Chunky-Monkey Banana Bread Granola

Need a healthy breakfast that is totally toteable?! Make a batch of this Chunky-Monkey Banana Bread Granola we've found a different way to make it chunky: with almond butter and bananas".

Ingredients

1 cup rolled oats.

1 cup pecans.

1 cup buckwheat groaties.

1 cup walnuts.

2 tablespoons chia seeds.

1 teaspoon cinnamon.

1 teaspoon vanilla powder.

1/4 teaspoon salt.

1/4 cup almond butter.

1 large ripe banana, mashed (about 1/2 cup).

1/4 cup coconut oil.

Instructions

1. Preheat the oven to 180ºC/350ºF/Gas Mark 4 and line a large baking tray with baking paper.

2. Add all ingredients to a large mixing bowl. Using a wooden spoon, mix all ingredients until everyday is nicely coated. Scoop onto the prepared baking tray and roughly flatten out. You still want to leave a few large chunky pieces.

3. Place in the oven and cook for 20 minutes, turning halfway. Once nicely browned, remove granola from the oven and allow to cool completely, this will make your clusters hold together better.

Note

Serve granola with full-fat natural or Greek yoghurt if you fancy

Sugar Free Snack – Turkey & Avocado Toasts

Ingredients – One serving

½ avocado, flesh only

Juice of ½ a lime

2-3 small slices ciabatta bread

50 grams turkey slices

Ground black pepper

2-3 cherry tomatoes, halved

Chili flakes – optional

Method

Mash the avocado with the lime juice in a bowl until you form a smooth paste. Toast the ciabatta and then spread with mashed avocado. Top with turkey and finish with ground black pepper. Eat while still warm. Garnish with a few cherry tomatoes to pump up the nutritional content of this great-tasting snack. I love to spice this snack up with a hearty sprinkling of dried chili flakes. Try it – you'll love them too!

Nutritional breakdown

Calories 208

Fat 11 grams

Carbohydrate 12 grams

Sugar 3.1 grams

Protein 15 grams

Fiber 2 grams

Zucchini pizza bites

Ingredients

1 medium zucchini – sliced lengthways

1 tablespoon tomato paste

50 grams grated mozzarella

25 grams finely chopped bacon or ham

6 cherry tomatoes, sliced

Method

Take the zucchini slices and place them on a baking tray. Pop them under a pre-heated grill and cook until they begin to brown. Remove from the grill, turn them over and spread the slices with the tomato paste. Sprinkle the slices with the grated cheese and bacon/ham and then cover with the sliced tomato. Place the slices back under the grill and cook until the cheese begins to turn brown. Remove and serve immediately.

Nutritional breakdown

Calories 305

Fat 15.2 grams

Carbohydrate 17.6 grams

Sugar 11.1 grams

Protein 25.1 grams

Fiber 4.2 grams

What Now?

If you really want to rid yourself of sugar cravings, lose weight and get healthier, a good way to do it is to avoid added sugars. Remember, sugar that is found naturally in plants that you eat is usually okay, although you should try to limit super-sweet fruit like dried fruits and dates.

Take it one day at a time. Focus on eating until you're satisfied and not stuffed whenever you're hungry. Get enough hydration, exercise, and sunshine and you'll kick that sugar habit to the curb in no time.

Sugar Health Effects

A 2003 WHO technical report provided evidence that high intake of sugary drinks (including fruit juice) increased the risk of obesity by adding to overall energy intake. The 'empty calories' argument states that a diet high in added sugar will reduce consumption of foods that contain essential nutrients.

Obesity and metabolic syndrome

By itself, sugar is not a factor causing obesity and metabolic syndrome, but rather – when over-consumed – is a component of unhealthy dietary behavior. Controlled trials showed that overconsumption of sugar-sweetened beverages increases body weight and body fat, and that replacement of sugar by artificial sweeteners reduces weight. Other studies showed correlation between refined sugar ("free sugar") consumption and the onset of diabetes, and negative correlation with the consumption of fiber.

Cardiovascular disease

From systematic reviews published in 2016, there is no evidence that sugar intake at normal levels increases the risk of cardiovascular diseases. Sugar, particularly fructose, does not have unique effects causing injury to the cardiovascular system, but rather excess total energy intake increases risk of cardiovascular and metabolic diseases.

Addiction

Reviews published in 2014 and 2016 suggest that sugar addiction does not occur in humans.

Hyperactivity

Some studies report evidence of causality between refined sugar and hyperactivity. The 2003 WHO report suggests that inconclusive evidence for sugar as a cause of hyperactivity is expected when studies do not control for intake of free sugars versus unrefined sugars.

Tooth decay

The 2003 WHO report stated that "Sugars are undoubtedly the most important dietary factor in the development of dental caries".For tooth decay, there is "convincing evidence from human intervention studies, epidemiological studies, animal studies and experimental studies, for an association between the amount and frequency of free sugars intake and dental caries" while other sugars (complex carbohydrate) consumption is normally associated with a lower rate of dental caries. Also, studies have shown that the consumption of sugar and starch have different impacts on oral health, with the ingestion of starchy foods and fresh fruit being associated with lower incidence of dental caries.

Alzheimer's disease

Claims have been made of a sugar–Alzheimer's disease connection, but there is inconclusive evidence that cognitive decline is related to dietary fructose or overall energy intake

Recommended dietary intake

The World Health Organization recommends that both adults and children reduce the intake of free sugars to less than 10% of total energy intake. A reduction to below 5% of total energy intake brings additional health benefits, especially in what regards dental caries (cavities in the teeth). These recommendations were based on the totality of available evidence reviewed regarding the relationship between free sugars intake and body weight and dental caries. Free sugars include monosaccharides and disaccharides added to foods and beverages by the manufacturer, cook or consumer, and sugars naturally present in honey, syrups, fruit juices and fruit juice concentrates.

On May 20, 2016 the U.S. Food and Drug Administration announced changes to the Nutrition Facts panel displayed on all foods, to be effective by July 2018. New to the panel is a requirement to list "Added sugars" by weight and as a percent of Daily Value (DV). For vitamins and minerals the intent of DVs is to indicate how much should be consumed. For added sugars, the guidance is that 100% DV should not be exceeded. 100% DV is defined as 50 grams. For a person consuming 2000 calories a day, 50 grams, the amount to not exceed, is the same as 200 calories, and thus 10% of total calories – same guidance as the World Health Organization. To put this into context, most 12 ounce (335 mL) cans of soda contain 39 grams of sugar. In the United States, a recently published government survey on food consumption reported that for men and women ages 20 and older the average total sugar intakes – naturally occurring in foods and added – were, respectively, 125 and 99 g/day.